POWER OVER AUTOIMMUNE

Take Back Control of Your Condition and Live the Life You Were Always Meant to Live

Gregg Haven M.D.

DEDICATION

I DEDICATE THIS BOOK TO ALL OF YOU WHO
WANTS TO OVERCOME THIS DISEASE AND
LIVE A HEALTHY AND HAPPY LIFE.

Dear Treasured Reader,

Thank you so much for purchasing a copy of "Power Over Autoimmune" and congratulate you for taking the first step to take control of your autoimmune problem. I hope you get exactly what you were looking for in this book and so much more.

I would also like to make a formal request to you to help me in getting the word out on this book to others looking for solutions to the autoimmune problem.

One way you could do that is if you'd be so kind to leave a review on the platform that you purchased or downloaded this book from if you liked/enjoyed this book at any point in your reading.

Additionally, if you have any topics and suggestions that you would like included in the book to help solve any problems/queries that were not addressed, do feedback in the review as well.

Thank You Once Again!

CONTENTS

INTRODUCTION

The number of US citizens that are diagnosed with chronic conditions is on the rise. It has been predicted that close to half of the population will be diagnosed with some kind of chronic condition by 2030. This could mean several things. First, more people are becoming sick early in their life. Second, it is estimated that by the year 2044 the cost of Medicaid and Medicare to treat these problems will rise to more than all the taxes that the government collects. What's even worse is that the most common conditions are grouped together as autoimmune diseases, which is where the body, while it is trying to heal itself, is attacking itself instead.

How should we handle this then? The answer begins at home and not in a doctor's office. Health begins where you live, in the kitchen where you cook, and the places where you eat.

Science has told us that the foods that most of us grew up on and taught to enjoy our whole life, and foods that many still eat to this day, are actually causing us to be sick. These types of foods include wheat products, commercially processed fats, dairy, and sugar. Once you start to understand this, you are well on your way to changing your relationship with what you eat, and you will start to feel better. That is what you are going to find in this book.

Traditional medicine is partly to blame for the problems that people are facing health-wise. When doctors said to fight obesity with a low-fat diet, they turn their patients to a diet full of whole grain pasta, margarine, and bread. Yet over the past few years, it has been found that the advice was wrong because the opposite tends to happen. Low-fat is not the way to cure the obesity problem; it was the main cause.

Now they have found that consuming foods high in good fats will make you think. Sugar causes you to become fat, and the body converts flour products into sugar, which is one of the biggest contributors to the epidemic.

The way that they grind flour now, and the way that it is grown, make wheat has a lot more starch than the kind of wheat that our ancestors consumed. The average loaf of whole wheat bread contains more sugar than sugar. Two slices of whole wheat bread will raise your blood sugar more than a candy bar would.

If you are one of the many people in the world that know that that just does not feel right, but you are not sure as to why, then this book will help you. The information in this book takes you beyond the traditional health system and provides you with information that will help. You will learn how to use strategies that will help you change your behaviors so that you will start feeling better and will lose weight and regain energy.

This will not be an easy journey and will take a lot of effort. You will have to pick the solutions that work the best for you, and you can tweak them to fit your lifestyle the best. Not all of these solutions will suit you, and if you can make a particular lifestyle change, that is perfectly all right.

PART 1:
THE AUTOIMMUNE
PROBLEM

CHAPTER 1: ORIGINATION

An autoimmune disease is a condition that happens when the body has an unusual immune response to a healthy body part. At the moment, there are 80 known types of autoimmune diseases. Almost any part of the body can be affected by this problem. Many of the most common systems are feeling tired and having a low-grade fever. Most of the times, these symptoms will come and go.

The primary cause of this problem is unknown. There are some of this disease that is hereditary, like lupus, and there are some cases where it can be triggered by an infection or environmental factor.

Some of the most common autoimmune diseases are systemic lupus, rheumatoid arthritis, psoriasis, multiple sclerosis, inflammatory bowel disease, Graves' disease, type 1 diabetes, and celiac disease.

In the US, about 24 million people are affected by an autoimmune disease. Women are more often affected than men. This disease will typically start during adulthood. The first of these diseases were described during the early 1900s. A disease has to answer to Witebsky's postulates to be classified as autoimmune. This includes:

- The disease is incurable
- There is genetic evidence of clustering with other diseases
- Circumstantial clinical clues
- Evidence found in the disease reproduction in animals
- Direct signs of disease-causing antibody or T-

lymphocyte white blood cells

While doctors and scientists still seem unsure as to what causes these diseases, new research may have discovered a way to diagnose the disease better and improve treatments.

A group of scientists from Yale School of Medicine, Broad Institute of MIT and Harvard, and UC San Francisco came up with new mathematical tools to look more deeply into existing DNA. By doing so, they have found how variations, when inherited, may contribute to disease.

By using their new method to analyze data from research done on 21 different diseases, they were able to deepen the understanding of how genetics plays a role in many different disorders. They were also able to find certain immune cells that were responsible for diseases.

They looked at 39 large-scale studies known as GWAS, which means Genome-Wide Association

Studies. This GWAS enlists many participants for the study to identify blocks of DNA where genetic variants may implicate a risk factor for diseases. However, this data has not actually pointed to altered proteins.

Instead, they found that the DNA variation does not reside within the genes. New research has found the presence of certain genetic variants in various diseases changes gene activity patterns in a certain way that affects the function of the immune system.

They have concluded that there are 300 to 400 known genetic variants that work together to cause autoimmune disease, which is spread through the human genome. These genes are often located close to regions that play an important part in regulating immune function.

They now know there are two basic types of genetic diseases. One is where there is a particular mutation in a certain gene, like when it comes to muscular dystrophy, which causes the problem. But the majority of autoimmune diseases originate from a complex blend of typically helpful genetic variants that everybody has, but for some, it results in illness.

Here are five leading causes of autoimmune disease:

1. Hygiene theory: This country, along with others, have sanitized the environment with antibacterial soaps and many other hygiene habits that have resulted in a reduction in how much we are exposed to dirt and microbes that the body is taught how to fight. This is causing an imbalance in the immune system.

2. Microbiome theory: The gut bacteria regulate how the immune system works and is being destroyed by medications and antibiotics, as well as processed foods.

3. Leaky gut syndrome: The lining of the digestive tract houses 70% of the immune system. When the cells within this lining become damaged,

the lining may become permeable. This will cause the immune system to start reacting to medication, foods, and many other things. This means that the immune system is always ready to respond.

4. Vitamin D deficiency: In some studies, this has been linked to autoimmune diseases.

5. Stress: When you have high levels of cortisol, it can affect the way the immune system works.

CHAPTER 2: MYTHS AND FACTS

The following will cover several myths that seem to revolve around autoimmune diseases.

Myth 1 – These disorders cannot be changed

There may be a genetic part to autoimmune disorders, but it has been discovered through epigenetics that gene expression can be modified. For a disorder to happen, there has to be something that triggers it, but with intestinal healing and diet you can switch these genetic problems off and fix your immune system.

Myth 2 – Symptoms will not go away without medications

Many doctors will dismiss the importance of nutrition. Because of this, patients are prescribed drugs for their disorders. Instead of having to take medicines that suppress the immune system, supplements and food can support and strengthen it while healing the gut. Medications are not the only option.

Myth 3 – The side effects of medications are not important

The side effects of the drugs used for autoimmune problems are common, happen often, and are disruptive. This could mean headaches, high blood pressure, weight gain, insomnia, or any other possibility.

Myth 4 – Better gut health and digestion does not affect autoimmune disorders

The digestive system and the immune system may be two different parts of the body, but if you ignore the gut, you can cause problems. Most of the immune system is in the gut, so it is important to focus on the digestive system and heal the gut.

Myth 5 – The environment does not matter

Only 25% of your chances of developing an autoimmune disease comes from genetics. That means the other 75% is environmental. You can affect your body's response by shifting areas of your life so you can support your immune system and create a better life.

Myth 6 – Having a gluten-free diet will not change your autoimmune disorder

Going gluten-free? That is only a fad that people want to cash in on. Our ancestors have been consuming wheat for thousands of years, but all of sudden it has turned out not to be healthy for us, why?

This is what the majority of people believe when it comes to gluten and our health, and a lot of conventional practitioners do not view it any differently. If you were to mention to your doctor that you were concerned about what gluten is doing to you, and more likely than not she or he is going to say two things: "We can run a test and see if you suffer from celiac disease" and "Do you suffer from digestive problems? No? Then there's no reason for you to worry about gluten."

Thinking that gluten does not affect autoimmune conditions is probably one of the most dangerous myths that a person can have about an autoimmune disorder. Getting rid of this myth is probably of the best things that can help people with autoimmune disorders.

Myth 7 – You are doomed to have a poor quality of life if you have an autoimmune disease

"I was informed by my doctor that, over time, I would start to get weaker and weaker."

"I had to decide to tell my son he cannot bring over the grandkids because I just cannot take the risk of getting sick."

"The pain can become so severe that I have problems taking a walk with my husband."

These are some of the challenges that a person who suffers from an autoimmune disease can expect to happen, sometimes frequently, but it does not mean that they are inevitable. With conventional medicine, they will end up counseling you into accepting a poor quality of life because they will make you think that your likely outcome with your condition. I'm here to let you know that this is not all inevitable.

Myth 8 – It has to do with your immune system, so there is nothing that you can do about it

Regular medical doctors will treat the autoimmune condition by helping to suppress the immune system and medicate the symptoms. If you look at The Myers Way, it will treat the autoimmune condition by helping to strengthen the immune system, which involves supporting and cleansing the gut.

CHAPTER 3: IS THERE A CURE?

A little ten-year-old girl who enjoyed riding horses went to the doctor with a severe autoimmune disease. Her joints were swollen, her skin was inflamed, her face was swollen, her immune system was hurting her whole body: her red and white blood cells, liver, blood vessels, joints, skin, muscles. She was unable to make a fist. The tip ends of her toes and fingers were cold because of Raynaud's disease that was inflaming her blood vessels. She was losing her hair, tired, and miserable. She had to take elephant dose of steroids intravenously every three weeks section she could stay alive. She also had to take a chemo drug, methotrexate, acid blockers, aspirin, and prednisone to shut her immune system down.

Despite the medication, she did not see any results, and her tests stayed abnormal. Her regular doctors wanted to add more immune-suppressing drugs to the medication she already took. They wanted to put her on a drug that increases the risk of cancer and death from infections because it keeps the immune system from being able to fight off infections. She was not willing to accept this, so she went to get a second opinion.

Two months her first visit with the new doctor, where he figured out the underlying cause of her problems, she has quit consuming sugar, dairy, and gluten and began taking supplements, she was symptom-free. In a little less than a year, she was healthy, and her test came back normal, and she did not have to take her medications anymore.

Because of this true story, what does it mean for autoimmune disease research and how doctors approach the treatment of them? While there may be many of these diseases, they have something in common; the body starts attacking itself. So there may not be a drug that can cure these diseases, but there is of course another way to treat them.

It used to be that medical discoveries start with a physician who has observed their patients' disease and their response to treatment. Doctors would report their findings to coworkers or would publish them as a case study. Now a lot of these case studies wind up being dismissed as a story and have ended up becoming irrelevant. People now look towards random controlled trial. The problem is this dismisses thousands of patients and doctors' experiences.

These fundamental discoveries can take years to be translated into regular practice. This prevents many people from accessing new therapies that they need now. The determining fact on figuring out a new approach is what the risk and benefits are to the patient.

Besides the use of antibiotics for infections and treating trauma, most medicine today tries to suppress, cover up, block, or otherwise interfere with the human body's natural workings. Doctors will not try to fix the underlying problems in the first place.

Instead, we need to ask why is the body having problems and how can it be fixed?

Functional medicine is beginning to look at things like this. This is a hidden movement that is starting to sweep the globe, and it focuses on the cause and not the symptoms. It is based on understanding the way the genes interact with the environment, and it goes past simply treating things based on labels.

For the little girl we talked about earlier, her doctors' response to her illness was to suppress the immune system, which left her open to psychiatric illness, muscle wasting, osteoporosis, infection, and cancer. But then she found somebody that asked why. He did not look at the name of the disease, but instead why the disease was there, where it started, and how to locate the cause and create a balance to her immune system.

The immune system will respond to some problem, like an allergen, toxin, or microbe, and then will go out of control. Figuring out that trigger and getting rid of it is crucial.

When the little girl's new doctor talked to her, he found that there were a lot of possible triggers. She had been exposed to Stachybotrys, a toxic mold, that was in her house. Her mother, while pregnant, had worked in limestone pits which exposed her to fluoride. She had her vaccination before 1999, which was when thimerosal was taken out of vaccines. She also took a flu shot that contains thimerosal every year. Thimerosal contains mercury, which is an immune toxin. This problem was increased by what she ate. She regularly consumed sushi and tuna, and loads of sugar, dairy, and gluten. The year before her getting sick, she had many doses of antibiotics.

The new doctor performed tests, and he found her liver function and muscle enzyme tests showed lots of damage. There were a lot of autoimmune antibodies, which means that the levels the body was attacking itself were extremely high. Markers of inflammation were also high. Her white and red blood cell count was low, as well as her vitamin D. She also has high levels of mercury; her level was 33, the normal is less than three.

After her visit to the new doctor, he placed her on an elimination diet to get rid of all the possible triggers. She got rid of gluten, sugar, and dairy. He also prescribed her a multivitamin; one that contained evening primrose oil, fish oil, folate, B12, and vitamin D. He also prescribed her Nystatin, which is a nonabsorbed anti-fungal, to treat yeast. She was also given NAC (N-Acetyl Cysteine) to help her liver. The doctor also told her to stop the intravenous steroids, calcium channel blocker, and the acid blocker she had been taken.

Two months later the rash was completely gone. Her hair was growing back, and her joint pain was gone. Autoimmune markers have also improved. Her inflammation level, liver function, and muscle enzymes were normal again.

At her next visit, she was given probiotics to help her digestive function and gut health. continuing to work also gave her DMSA (Dimercaptosuccinic Acid) to remove the mercury from her cells and tissues. She was also given herbs to help her adrenal gland and so that she could stop taking prednisone.

After seven months, all of her tests were perfect, including her white blood cells count. Mercury levels had decreased from 33 to 16. By month 11, her mercury levels were at 11. She did not have to take any of her medications and was feeling normal, happy, and could ride a horse again.

Some people may be able to dismiss this as a spontaneous remission, or claim that the testing was unconventional, or the treatment unproven. But there is a shimmer of hope that this could work, and it can help to recover from a devastating and debilitating disease.

This little girl's story is not one in a million. This approach of figuring out and getting rid of triggers for a disease like hidden allergens, toxins, or microbes, and supporting how the body functions with herbs and nutrients and "pro" drugs are more than just an idea that has to be proven. This is a movement that thousands of practitioners are using. It is an approach that has already helped thousands of patients around the world. Doctors have the knowledge and the methods, so why not apply them?

CHAPTER 4: HISTAMINE INTOLERANCE

Do you ever have unexplained anxiety or headaches? Do you have irregular menstrual cycles? When you drink red wine, does your face flush? Do you experience a runny nose or itchy tongue when you eat eggplants, bananas, or avocados? If you said yes to any one of these questions, then you may have histamine intolerance.

Histamine is a chemical that works with the immune system, central nervous system, and digestion. It is a neurotransmitter that communicates messages from the body up to the brain. It also works with stomach acid, which breaks down the food in the stomach.

You are probably most familiar with what histamine is as it relates to the immune system. If you have seasonal allergies or a food allergy, you probably know that antihistamine drugs such as Benadryl, Zyrtec, or Allegra will give you fast relief. The reason for this is because histamine's job within the body is to create an immediate inflammatory response. It's a red flag for the immune system and tells your body that there is a potential risk.

Histamine will swell or dilate the blood vessels so that the white blood cells can get to problems and fix it. The buildup of histamine is what causes you to have a headache, and leaves you feeling miserable, flushed, and itchy. This is a natural immune response, but if your body does not break down histamine correctly, you may end up developing histamine intolerance.

Since histamine travels through the blood, it can

affect your cardiovascular system, brain, skin, lungs, and gut causing many different problems making it hard to diagnose.

Symptoms of histamine intolerance can include:

- Tissue swelling

- Fatigue

- Hives

- Abnormal menstrual cycle

- Difficulty breathing, nasal congestion, sneezing

- Flushing

- Abdominal cramps

  - Vomiting, nausea

- Anxiety

- Difficulty regulating body temp

- Accelerated heart rate or arrhythmia

- Dizziness or vertigo

- Hypertension

- Easily awoken, difficulty falling asleep

- Migraines or headaches

Things that can cause high levels of histamine mean are histamine-rich foods, diamine oxidase deficiency, fermented alcohol, GI bleeding leaky gut, bacterial overgrowth, and allergies.

Besides the histamine that the body naturally produces, some foods contain histamine or block the enzyme that helps to break histamine down.

Once histamine has been formed, it will either be stored or broken down by a particular enzyme. In the central nervous system, histamine is broken down typically by histamine N-methyltransferase, while in the digestive tracts it will be broken down by diamine oxidase. Even though both enzymes work to break down histamine, it has been found that DAO (Diamine Oxidase) is the primary enzyme that works to breaks down ingested histamine. If you have a deficiency in DAO, you will probably suffer from histamine intolerance.

You can get tested for histamine intolerance to

make sure if you suffer from it. The first you can do on your own: elimination and reintroduction. Start by removing foods high in histamine for 30 days and start reintroducing them one at a time. You can get a blood test that will check your histamine and DAO levels. If you have a high ratio of histamine to DAO, then you may be ingesting a lot of histamines, and your DAO is too low to break it down.

If you can get a blood test, you can start eating a diet that is low in histamine and start taking a DAO supplement with each meal. If you notice that your symptoms go away, then you may have low DAO.

To treat histamine intolerance, get rid of foods high in histamine from one to three months. Start taking a DAO supplement, which you will take two pills at every meal. However, remember, consult your doctor before taking any supplement. The most important thing is to figure out the cause of your histamine intolerance. If you take a medication that is causing this intolerance, talk with your doctor to see about getting you off these drugs. The most common cause is gluten intolerance and SIBO, which will cause leaky gut. If that is your problem, then you can heal your gut, and you will not have to eliminate foods, and you will not have to take DAO.

If you find that you do suffer from histamine intolerance, the good news is that you may not have to stay away from histamine foods for forever. This is just a short-term fix until DAO or histamine levels get back to normal. Depending on you, you could find that you can handle some foods better than others, so make sure you stay optimistic.

PART 2:
THE SOLUTION

CHAPTER 5: BEGIN WITH THE GUT

While it is easy to overlook the health of the gastrointestinal system (GI), it still contains ten times healthier bacteria than any other part of the body. It helps to promote elimination and healthy digestion, supports metabolism, and protects us from infection. Unfortunately, most people had inadequate beneficial bacteria and took many damaging bacteria, and they lack diversity. This is mainly due to a bad diet, but may be caused from:

- Current body and health composition – poor disease status

- Inadequate bacterial acquisition at birth – C-section, parent gut health, mother's diet during pregnancy, transition from breast milk to solid food

- Environment toxins – BPA, arsenic, herbicides, PCBs, pesticides
- Chronic stress
- Over-medicating – antacids, antidepressants, NSAIDs, birth control, antibiotics

All of this will lead to unbalanced gut flora, and this increases the chance of permeability. This is because the same things that hurt out gut flora and compromise the gut barrier; while infections and harmful bacteria can prosper can do the same.

This is caused by the fact that even though the gut is inside the body, it is really an external organ that's role is to keep harmful substances out of the body. So if the barrier is becoming compromised, foreign molecules can pass into the bloodstream, and problems can start. The body will then launch into an immune response for protection, but ends up hurting your tissues and organs. Recent research has found that leaky gut is connected to hundreds of medical conditions including:

- Chronic kidney disease
- Dermatitis
- Schizophrenia
- Parkinson's
- Allergies and asthma
- Type 1 diabetes
- Chronic fatigue
- Lupus
- Multiple sclerosis
- Social anxiety and depression
- IBD
- Autism, ADHA, and Tourette's
- Rheumatoid arthritis
- Fibromyalgia

This tends to be where some will get upset and quit listening. This because if it is true, which research suggest it is, the underlying problem to your health was caused by you, since your upset gut was caused by what you did; whether exposing yourself to bad things, eating certain foods, or over medicating.

But the thing is, it is not actually your fault.

The only thing you are guilty of is listening to "experts" and choosing the best choices you were given. These are the same options that everybody else was faced with. Unfortunately for you, or your relatives, may not have as much genetic protection as others. Or you just did not start out with a strong shot from the get-go.

This should give you hope. It means that you can change your performance and health. If you are dealing with or taking care of someone who is dealing with a gastrointestinal problem, mental disorder, or neurological condition, you can potentially change your life.

A little honesty here though, there is no guarantee that it will help, but the evidence makes us believe that this kind of problems does start in the gut. Helping the gut out can give you improvements.

While not every disease may be because of leaky gut, and not everybody has leaky gut, but evidence shows us that an old hypothesis is not quackery. So there is really no reason why you shouldn't be doing something to promote gut health and improve the integrity of the gut lining.

To help heal your gut, you can follow this four-part system known as the 4 R's:

Remove

Get rid of all the bad. The goal here is to eliminate the things that negatively affect your gut like drugs, caffeine, alcohol, infections, and inflammatory foods.

Inflammatory foods can include sugar, eggs, soy, corn, dairy, and gluten because they can lead to sensitivities. An elimination diet is a good starting point to figure out the foods that cause you the most problems. This is where you remove foods for a couple of weeks and then start to add them back in and to notice how your body responds.

Infections may be caused by bacteria, yeast, or parasites. It's important to get a comprehensive stool analysis to determine your levels of good bacteria and possible infections that you could have. Getting rid of the infections may mean treatments with antifungal supplements, antifungal medication, anti-parasite medication, herbs, and antibiotics, if entirely necessary.

Replace

Add in good. Start adding in the things that are essential for proper absorption and digestion that may have become depleted by aging, diseases, drugs, or diet. This could include bile acids, hydrochloric acid, and digestive enzymes that are needed for proper digestion.

Reinoculate

Restoring the good bacteria to reestablish a good balance of beneficial bacteria is important. This can be done by taking a probiotic that contains good bacteria like lactobacillus and bifidobacteria species. 25 to 100 billion units each day is a good range to go for. A prebiotic supplement or eating foods that are high in soluble fiber is also important.

Repair

Give your system the nutrients that it needs to help fix the gut itself. An excellent supplement for that is L-glutamine, which is an amino acid that helps the gut wall lining. Other types of nutrients are vitamin E, A, and C, Omega-3 fish oils, and zinc, along with herbs like aloe vera and slippery elm.

No matter the problems you are facing, the 4 R's can help to heal up your gut. Lots of inflammatory and chronic illnesses respond positively to this in just a short amount of time.

CHAPTER 6: CHOOSING THE BEST FOODS

Most autoimmune diseases are often treated with immunosuppressive medications, which will only cause bigger risks for the body. The good thing is, more research has found that a dietary change can lower the symptom severity, stop disease progression, and may even keep the problem from ever starting.

Omega-3 fats can reduce inflammation. Average Americans today will have a diet that has an unbalanced proportion of omega-6 and omega-3 fatty acid. Ideally, the body needs more omega-3 fatty acids because they provide an anti-inflammatory effect. Omega-6 fatty acids are important if they are in higher concentrations in the diet from processed foods, and with large amounts of vegetable oils, it can cause an increase in molecules which can cause inflammation.

Some individuals that suffer from various autoimmune diseases have seen an improvement in their symptoms by taking a fish oil supplement. People that have rheumatoid arthritis had a 73% decrease in drug treatment. Patients that had Crohn's disease had a 60% reduction in their relapse rate.

Fatty acids help to decrease an immune system that caused inflammation. Fatty acids can suppress the antibodies that cause an immune system alarm for defense and contributes to improving pathways of the cells that cause inflammation.

If you tend to experience symptom flare-ups without any reason, oxalates may cause inflammation. If you can detect that oxalates are causing your autoimmune response, then you can heal yourself quicker.

Oxalates are compounds that naturally occur in nature that is found in protein alternatives like some veggies and fruits, nuts, grains, and soy. Some of these foods can be added to a healthy diet, if you have an unhealthy gut you can experience oxidative stress, nutrient deficiency, and chronic inflammation that can damage the body.

Antioxidants can help reduce inflammation. If there is an increase in antioxidants, it can decrease oxidative stress, which causes tissue damage, and that means it is directly correlated with the reduction of inflammation, autoimmune disease, and chronic illness. A study discovered that a diet that was supplemented with antioxidants and was lower in caloric and fat intake delayed the start of Lupus symptoms by stimulating the immune system.

Antioxidants will help the brain from oxidative stress which is known to cause loss of cognitive function and aging. Maintaining a healthy mind and gut interaction is essential for healthy vitality and aging.

Vitamins that provide antioxidants have anti-inflammatory properties that inhibit cytokine activity for diseases that are autoimmune, which are what signals an inflammatory response in cells. Herbs that have high levels of antioxidants, like curcumin which comes from turmeric, have shown to have the same anti-inflammatory response as synthetic drugs like aspirin.

B-12, folate, and B-6 all have antioxidant properties. Vitamin B-6 has been found to inhibit macrophages from taking over foreign matters that are associated with autoimmune problems. A deficiency in B-6 has been shown to correlate with increased sensitivity to oxalates contained in food.

A person with the MTHFR gene (Methylenetetrahydrofolate reductase) mutation has a lower ability to produce important antioxidant glutathione. This is crucial for immune modulation and detoxification. Small makes them at a higher risk of developing chronic inflammatory diseases and autoimmune problems.

Stay away from nightshades. This includes any pepper, white potato, and tomatoes and they help an unhealthy autoimmune response. Nightshades will increase calcium deposits within tissues which can cause chronic inflammation which will cause more problems and health consequences.

Damage to the liver and kidneys can cause autoimmune diseases like diabetes and rheumatoid arthritis. Not all people have a negative response to nightshades. However, people that have autoimmune problems will struggle with the foods.

Here are some nutritional tips:

- Drink purified water
- Buy organic. Toxins found in pesticides can destroy gut health

- Avoid foods that do not come from nature

- Switch vegetable oils to cold pressed oils like coconut and olive

- Eliminate refined sugars

- Commit to prebiotic and probiotic supplements

- Get rid of coffee and switch to organic teas

Let's touch on that last point, coffee. Coffee tends to affect people with an autoimmune disorder negatively. Coffee comes from a seed and is not recommended when it comes to an autoimmune diet. Seeds and nuts typically cause the least problems, so you may be able to add them back in.

For somebody with gluten intolerance or celiac disease, coffee can be harmful to them. Coffee is a cross-reactive food to gluten, which means that some bodies will view coffee the same as gluten.

Coffee will also overstimulate the adrenal glands which cause an increase in adrenal fatigue. People will get into the habit of use caffeine as their energy source, which gives short-term benefits but long-term problems. Decaf is not really any better than caffeinated because of the chemicals that are used to get rid of the caffeine.

Some good alternatives to coffee are rooibos tea, herbal teas, ginger infusion, and bone broth.

CHAPTER 7: STRESS

Stress has a strong connection with many health problems such as autoimmune problems, insomnia, heart disease, diabetes, and obesity. Internal inflammation also plays a role in the release of stress hormones, adding to an imbalance. If stress levels are not fixed, then serious problems can happen over time. When you experience a fight or flight response, cortisol is released. Whenever we experience danger, no matter how insignificant, the body will go into survival mode. The body will signal the adrenal cortex to release cortisol. While we can feel the increase in adrenaline, your body will also experience:

- Increase in glucose production
- Certain cells will not respond to insulin

- Production of insulin is reduced

- Tissue growth and repair is stopped

  - Arteries narrow causing an increase in blood pressure

Mental stress leads to an increase of cortisol which can cause a chronic anti-inflammatory response. This can result in the degradation of the digestive tract wall which can cause inflammation causing more cortisol to be released. This means that stress is only going to cause more problems, especially if you suffer from an autoimmune disease.

Stress and anxiety are like a monster under the bed that steals a peaceful night's sleep of almost 70 million Americans. Things like anxiety sabotage confidence and turn the stomach into knots and hurt your overall well-being. Here are five tips to help you get your stress and anxiety under control.

1. Remind yourself that it will pass

Your boss wants a report on yesterday's work, the

baby is sick, and the laundry is piling up. Does any of this sound familiar? Nobody that is taking care of their own life is going to be completely stress-free, and too much is going to lead to difficulty breathing, upset stomach, dread, nervousness, and excessive worry. The first step to overcoming these feelings is to understand that you are going through something common and what is known as anxiety. Even though the negative emotion is uncomfortable, these feelings are going to pass. If you fight these feelings, it will cause worse emotions. If you accept them, you will notice that you start feeling better.

2. Start Self-Soothing

Imagine yourself walking through the woods, and you end up meeting a bear, or worse, your boss demanding a report. When faced with a situation like this, the body's sympathetic nervous system will trigger physiological changes. The breath quickens, adrenaline is released, and the heart starts to race.

This is supposed to help us escape life-threatening emergency. Except when the threat is only imagined, it causes an unnecessary response. You can use diaphragmatic breathing for relaxation. You cannot manually reduce your heart rate; you can use deep breathing techniques to lower your pulse rate.

Positive self-talk is another way to self-soothe. Instead of using the comments that you frequently say to yourself like "that was a stupid mistake," try using positive phrases. Try using, "I'm safe now," "I can make it through this," and other positive sayings.

Muscle relaxation is another great option. To do this, go through your body and tight and then release your muscles. play a major role in will help the stress to release from the muscles, helping you to relax.

3. Check your diet

The things that you consume plays a big part in your emotional state. Alcohol and caffeine-containing foods exacerbate anxiety and stress more than any other. Do not abruptly eliminate them though. This can cause withdrawal symptoms, which can cause more problems. It's best if you slowly reduce them.

4. Get moving

Most everybody understands that exercise is essential for good health. Over the past few decades, research has found that exercise can be more effective than any medication. Keeping a healthy, non-obsessive, regular exercise routine can help to increase energy levels, enhance self-esteem, improve mood, and reduce stress. When you are exercising, the body will release a chemical called endorphins which interact with brain receptors causing euphoric feelings and will lower physical pain.

5. Sleep more

Pretty much everybody will feel crabby when he or she do not get a good night's sleep. Inadequate sleep is a prevalent emotional problem, and it's hard to figure out which one came first: poor sleep or stress.

One study has shown that losing only a few hours of sleep can cause an increase in exhaustion, sadness, anger, and stress.

CHAPTER 8: REST

We touched on sleep in the last chapter, now let's look at why it is so important. A person cannot be completely healthy if they do not get enough sleep. As we are sleeping, the body repairs and maintains itself, which is important in maintaining health. Sleep keeps the organs working, improves immunity, gives us energy, boosts mood, helps with stress, and enhances mental clarity.

Sleep deprivation can have these effects on the body:

- Increased risk of death
- Systemic inflammation
- Mental and mood problems
- Cognitive decline

- Obesity and weight gain

- Impaired immunity

Even though we understand the importance of sleep, our culture is still willing to sacrifice sleep for productivity. Most everybody will force his or her body to stay up past sundown, which is the time when the body expects to go to bed. Along with devices like phones and computers, this all can mess up our balance of hormones that you need to maintain and induce sleep. Most people will miss the ideal time to go to bed, get a second wind, which will cause problems falling asleep. Another issue in our culture is that we do not let our self-get enough sleep. Most people get around six hours of sleep when we really need eight to nine. This causes you to wake up feeling unrefreshed and exhausted and need of coffee.

Getting a good night sleep seems to be difficult for the average person, so imagine the difficulty for a person with an autoimmune disease. The stress, pain, and depression that is associated with autoimmunity can make getting a full and good night sleep difficult. The body has more inflammation and repair that it is faced with every day, meaning that sleep is even more important to those with an autoimmune disease than an average person. Because it's so important, getting adequate rest should be an important part of managing your autoimmune disease.

Here are some tips that will help you to get a better night's sleep:

- Make use of stress-management tools throughout your day

- Reduce the amount of exposure you have to blue light right before you go to bed. Make sure that you turn off all screens a few hours before you go to sleep.

- Think about making your bedroom a technology-free zone. You may find it easier to sleep if you do not take your devices to bed with yours.

- Stay away from stimulants like sugar and caffeine before bed.

- Make your sleeping environment dark and comfortable. If you cannot get your room completely dark, you may want to get an eye mask or blackout curtains.

- Come up with a bedtime ritual. This could be anything. You could take a little walk after dinner, take a bath, and read a book before going to bed. Find a relaxing routine that you do every day so that your body can calm down and you will be able to slip off to sleep.

- Do not go to sleep with a full belly. Make sure you have a few hours after your last meal before you try to go to sleep. This will give you system adequate digestion time.

PART 3:
THE PREVENTION

CHAPTER 9: WHAT TO GET RID OF

We have looked at many of the reasons for autoimmune diseases, and I have given you some ways to reverse symptoms associated with these conditions and to balance the immune system.

Now let's look at the top triggers that can create flare-ups that will cause devastating symptoms. The following foods probably need to be removed from your diet. This goes for somebody with a full-blown disease like Hashimoto's, celiac, or Crohn's disease, or a common "autoimmune spectrum disorder" such as IBS or acne. You need to be aware of the possible landmines that can cause an inflammatory response.

1. Gluten

This "G" word is one of the proteins found in rye, spelled, barley, wheat, and many other grains. This protein has been linked to many different risks for autoimmunity.

There are a lot of doctors and people that believe you have to have celiac disease to be intolerant to gluten. When the lab results tell them they do not have celiac, the doctors say they do not need to cut out gluten. This kind of misinformation is what keeps people struggling with their autoimmune conditions.

For a lot of people that suffer from autoimmune problems, it does not take a piece of pasta or bread to cause problems. Food that was cross-contaminated with gluten can cause problems for them.

2. Gluten-free grains

Most people that have autoimmune problems will have already cut out gluten, but they will still consume rice, oats, and corn. As well-intentioned as this may be, this kind of grains is still just as damaging as gluten can be, and maybe even more so.

The proteins found in these ground are a lot like gluten, which is just like play Russian roulette for a person that suffers from an autoimmune condition. Similar to having a gluten sensitivity, these symptoms do not have to be gastrointestinal. Any sort of autoimmune symptom flare-up can happen when these grains are consumed.

Everybody is different, so it could be helpful that you run immunological blood tests to see the things that your body cross-reacts with.

3. Quinoa

One of the favorites within the health community is the pseudo-grain quinoa. They contain high levels of the protein saponin which can cause problems for the lining of the gut, which causes an immune response within the body. If you soak and rinse the quinoa, it can reduce its damaging effects to the gut, but for people with autoimmune conditions, it may not be enough.

4. Toxins

The environment is full of toxins that 100 years ago were unknown. Studies have found that these toxins play a part in autoimmune problems like autoimmune thyroiditis.

5. Sugar

It probably does not come as a surprise that sugar would be on this list, but this does not just include the stereotypical junk food. There are lots of "healthy" junk foods out there that are popular within the health community that can cause adverse effects to autoimmune problems.

Healthier sounding foods like agave nectar and organic turbinado sugar written on a food label may make it sound natural and earthy, but to your immune system sugar is still sugar.

6. Chocolate

This very yummy food can create a lot of damage to people that live with an autoimmune condition. Research has found that people who suffer from an autoimmune disease may be affected negatively by the consumption of chocolate.

7. Dairy

Casein is one of the main proteins that are found in milk, and many other dairy products may cause a trigger for inflammation within the body. Getting rid of the dairy proteins within clarified butter or ghee can give some people a safer alternative. Some autoimmune disorders can handle fermented dairies, such as kefir or grass-fed whole yogurt.

8. Nightshades

This plant group contains spices, goji berries, eggplants, potatoes, peppers, and tomatoes that contain alkaloids within their skin. These can cause the body to have an inflammatory response.

9. SIBO

SIBO stands for *small intestinal bacterial overgrowth*. This occurs when the normal bacteria that live in the large intestines start to travel to the small intestines. This can end up leading to many localized autoimmune spectrum conditions like acid reflux and IBS. Chronic SIBO may also result in leaky gut, which will cause more autoimmune problems through the entire body.

10. Weakened microbiome

Most of your immune system lives within what is called the microbiome. This is a highly sophisticated gut ecosystem that is made up of bacterial colonies. This microbiome is what controls, not only the immune system, but also the genetic expression, brain, and hormones.

Fungal, parasitic, and yeast infections can a be implicated in many autoimmune problems like MS and Parkinson's. It is important that you understand these symptoms do not have to show up as gastrointestinal.

11. Leaky gut syndrome

Functional medicine believes that an increase in the permeability of the gut lining is a precursor to developing autoimmunity. Everything else that I have mentioned can lead to a leaky gut. This means that leaky gut is also seen as a casual trigger, but the effect of this will proceed from an autoimmune condition.

When the gut is damaged, any undigested food proteins, as well as bacterial endotoxins, will be able to pass through the protective lining of the gut, which will cause an autoimmune reaction throughout the entire body.

Basically, you need to find what is your underlying personal trigger. This can help eliminate years of unnecessary suffering that a lot of autoimmune suffers have to go through. I cannot stress this enough; everybody is different, so you need to find what works before for your unique case.

CHAPTER 10: REDUCE INFLAMMATION

Chronic inflammation plays a huge role in many diseases, like Crohn's disease, autoimmune diseases, type-2 diabetes, as well as the three top killers: stroke, cancer, and heart disease. Research is looking into the line between brain disorders like dementia and Alzheimer's disease and inflammation. Diet, lifestyle change, and exercise are powerful tools to fight inflammation. Here are some ways you can get rid of inflammation.

Balance Omega Fats

People eat too many inflammations-causing omega-6 fats that are found in fast food, processed foods, vegetable oils like corn and sunflower and not eating enough inflammation-soothing omega-3 fats like olive oil, canola, walnuts, flaxseeds, tuna, and salmon. A diet high in omega-6s and low in omega-3s will increase inflammation in the body. To balance your omega fats, choose fresh, unprocessed food. Swap the sunflower or corn oil for canola or olive oil and load your plate with foods that are rich in omega-3s. If you eat one source of Omega-3s each day, you will be doing great things for inflammation. Omega-3s boost some proteins that slow down inflammation and reduce the number of proteins that cause inflammation. If you just cannot get four grams with food, ask about a supplement. Taking a fish-oil supplement each day will reduce inflammatory markers by about 14 percent.

Yoga

People who practiced 75 to 90 minutes of yoga twice a week have lower levels of interleukin-6 and Creactive protein (CRP). These are two inflammatory markers. Practicing yoga can reduce stress responses. Researchers think yoga benefits people because it minimizes stress-related changes.

Eat More Soy

Eating 25 grams of soy each day can reduce the risk of inflammation-driven cardiovascular disease. There can be results with consuming just half that amount. Lunasin, a peptide found in tofu and soymilk when combined with other soy protein, can quell inflammation. If you have hormone-sensitive conditions like endometriosis and breast cancer, ask your doctor before increasing your soy intake.

Get a Massage

A massage is more than a treat. It is all a part of being healthy. Getting a 45-minute massage can lower two essential inflammation-promoting hormones. Massages can decrease inflammatory substances by increasing how much disease-fighting white blood cells. It can reduce stress hormones. These results are seen after just one massage.

Limit Bad Fats

Trans-fatty acids are linked to an increase in body inflammation. Trans fats are found in foods like margarine, crackers, cookies, and fried foods. If the label says zero-gram trans-fat, it might still have about one-half gram per serving. If you eat more than one serving, you are eating several grams. Look for partially hydrogenated oil on the label. If you see this, it has trans fats. Cut back on saturated fats, too. Replace butter with olive oil and be choosy about proteins. Eat more lean proteins like plant-based proteins such as beans, white-meat poultry, and fish.

Eat Greens

Here is another reason to eat your greens, nuts, and whole grains: these foods are all rich in magnesium. Have your doctor check your magnesium level with a blood test. Most people who have high inflammation markers have low magnesium levels. Individuals who have conditions that are associated with inflammation, like diabetes and heart disease have low magnesium levels. Eating magnesium-rich foods will help to lower inflammation.

Get Rid of Stress

If you are easily frazzled, you are opening the door for inflammation. A study found that people who have strong emotional reactions to stress will have a greater increase in circulating interleukin-6 when stressed. Stress will increase the heart rate and blood pressure, and this makes your blood vessels work harder. You are pounding on them and causing damage. If too much damage happens, inflammation persists.

Get More Sleep

If you do not get a minimum of six hours of restful sleep every night, you are susceptible to inflammation. Getting less than six hours of sleep has been linked to increased levels of three key markers like fibrinogen, CRP, and interleukin-6.

Exercise

Eating right and losing some weight with exercise is a great way to lower your inflammation. Working out can decrease inflammation even if you do not lose any weight. Why? Exercising at 60 to 80 percent of your heart rate can lower the level of CRP which is a key inflammation marker. Think about taking a brisk walk where you can talk but not hold a full conversation.

Drink Green Tea

If coffee is your go-to beverage, you may not want to get rid of tea, especially green tea. Green tea is full of antioxidants that help to slow down inflammation. Researchers found that green tea can stop the oxidative stress and inflammation that results from it. People who drank 500 mg of green tea daily halved their stress levels.

CHAPTER 11: COMMON MISTAKES

Many people who have autoimmune disease manage their condition with exercise and diet. They stay away from foods that cause inflammation, take their medicines, and use natural remedies. Many people struggle with their illness daily. Here are some things that can make your disease worse without you even realizing it.

Eating Specific Foods

Most people's first thought is to eat organic and cleaner foods. Just because the food is labeled as organic does not mean you need to eat it.

Nightshades like peppers, potatoes, and tomatoes

can cause inflammation in people with an autoimmune disorder. Grains, dairy, and eggs can cause inflammation as well. These are hard to digest, and this causes flare-ups to your condition.

No Live Probiotics

People who have an autoimmune disease have imbalances of gut flora. This leads to a digestive condition like Candida. Be sure that fermented vegetables are part of your diet. Sauerkraut and kimchi are great sources of good bacteria as well as non-dairy kefirs and apple cider vinegar.

Heavy Metal Toxicity

This is common in soda cans, smoke, paint, personal hygiene products, and seafood. These are hard to stay away from.

Heavy metals are associated with different health conditions like autoimmune diseases. Heavy metal toxicity causes many symptoms like fatigue, paralysis, memory problems, chronic pain and other conditions.

Be sure you get tested for heavy metal toxicity if you have an autoimmune disorder. Getting rid of these metals could make a huge difference in your life.

No Live Enzymes

The body produces many different digestive enzymes but digesting foods can deplete your enzyme stores. Many diets do not replenish their depleted enzymes. Smoothies, fresh juices, and salads are a great place to begin promoting digestive health.

Other factors might contribute to making autoimmune conditions worse like prescription medicines, vitamin D deficiency, etc.

Fixing these issues might be the key to better health, even if they do not make your disease go away entirely.

PART 4: COMPLIMENT YOUR AUTOIMMUNE DISEASE WITH THESE STRATEGIES

CHAPTER 12: NUTRITION

Some common questions about Autoimmune Protocol are: should it be done alone or should it be layered with other diets like a low carb, Candida, SCD, GAPS, or low-FODMAP diets? This chapter will discuss the different diets. You should always consult your doctor before changing or adding anything to what your doctor has told you to do.

Low-Carb Diet

The low-carb diet has different versions, but the main distinction is if the number of carbs is enough to put a person into ketosis. This is when the body relies on ketones and glucose to supply energy to the body.

It is achieved by eating less than 25 grams of carbs each day. This is a relative number as some can produce ketosis by eating a higher number of carbs, others have to eat less. Many consider a diet that is between 50 and 100 grams of carbs each day a low-carb diet. Some say a low-carb diet is effective against neurological disorders and some cancers. Others have success with weight loss or regaining insulin sensitivity by eating a low-carb diet.

The Candida and SCD Diet

These diets have different protocols but share a pathogen-specific approach. Their purpose is to get rid of foods that feed the overgrowth in the gut like starches even those that are included in the autoimmune protocol such as tapioca, squash, and sweet potatoes, grains, milk, fruit juice, sweeteners, fruit, and other foods.

These can help eliminate symptoms for people who have overgrowths but neither can eliminate pathogens by themselves. If someone experiences these symptoms when eating certain foods, do not blindly go one of the different pathogen-specific diets. Test the diet, do not guess. Many who can help successful recover from overgrowths know which pathogen they are fighting. Some might need to be approached from different angles like probiotics, antifungals, herbal or prescription antibiotics. Work with someone who is experienced in this area.

These diets do not eliminate many allergens, and that is a problem for some who have autoimmunities like nightshades, dairy, and eggs.

GAPS Diet

This is similar to the Candida and SCD diet since it incorporates a specific pathogen approach, but it does pinpoint allergens and gut-healing nutrients. This diet contains well-cooked meat, broth, and vegetables for a certain amount of time until more foods are added one at a time to determine if they can be tolerated.

The first ones to be introduced are nuts, ghee, fermented dairy, egg yolks, probiotics, and fermented vegetables. This diet is used with neurological conditions and autism and has been used with different chronic health problems.

Low-FODMAP Diet

This diet gets rid of short-chain fermentable carbs that feed the overgrowth of bacteria in the gut. Many problems like cramps, gas, bloating, diarrhea, constipation, and IBS use this diet to get their digestive issues under control. All high-FODMAP foods are gotten rid of for several weeks and then reintroduced slowly to see how well the body will tolerate it.

The low-FODMAP has been used for people with Candida, SIBO, malabsorption, and other imbalances. It helps with symptoms of digestive overgrowth, it is not an autoimmune specific diet and includes some allergens like nightshades, nuts, and eggs. For people who suffer from these issues and cannot get them relieved by AIP (Autoimmune Protocol), adding a low-FODMAP for a couple of weeks could be helpful.

Low-FODMAP is effective when managing an overgrowth, is not effective by itself to treat an overgrowth. It needs to be layered with an AIP to be effective.

There is a lot of information about AIP, but other's journeys are not your journey. Take it one step at a time. Remember in time you will find out things about your health that will allow you to make progress but it might not happen suddenly.

It is advisable for people who have an autoimmune disorder to supplement with minerals and vitamins.

Vitamin D

The best source of vitamin D is sunshine. It can be enhanced by other means. The immune system is impacted by vitamin D within your system.

This vitamin gets converted into a hormone known

as calcitriol. This will turn on an antibacterial protein and defense against any unrecognized invaders.

It is important to prevent an overreaction to these visitors or the body's cells. If you have an autoimmune disorder, ask your doctor to test your vitamin D level. If you are deficient, your system might not be properly functioning.

Vitamin A

Vitamin A is valuable to our diets. It is called the anti-infective vitamin since it is needed for the immune system to function normally.

It can do this by maintaining the mucous cells that are barriers to germs that are trying to invade our bodies. It helps to produce white blood cells that are vital to our immune system.

Vitamin A is needed for the immune system, but large amounts are not needed. Your body can get vitamin A from animal or plant sources. It is necessary for the body to metabolize vitamin D effectively.

Vitamin B6

This vitamin group has functions within the immune system. People who are deficient in vitamin B6 have decreased the production of white blood cells and interleukin-2.

Balance is important with all B complex vitamins since many are interdependent. Just like vitamin A, you just need a little amount of B6. Your body does not make this vitamin, so a very healthy diet or supplements are needed to get it.

Antioxidants

These are a group of compounds that neutralize or destroy free radicals in the body. They protect against oxidative damage to cells that are caused by aging or exposure to toxic substances or pollutants.

Inflammation is common with autoimmune disease, but do not underestimate the problems of oxidative stress.

Within an immune response, the production of free

radicals increases. This can cause oxidative stress. Most of the damage in autoimmune disease is caused by free radical damage to tissues and cell membranes.

Fish oil is a great supplement for people who suffer from an autoimmune disorder. Fish oil contains vitamin E that acts as an antioxidant when you combine it with selenium and vitamin C.

Antioxidants are found in healthy food like vegetables and fruits. The most effective ones are selenium, CoQ10, grape seed-skin extract, beta-carotene, green tea extract, vitamin E, and vitamin C.

Fish oils contain omega-3 fatty acids like DHA and EPA. These can regulate the immune system.

These have been successful in helping conditions like rheumatoid arthritis, multiple sclerosis, lupus erythematosus, Crohn's disease, and arthritis.

DHEA

This is a pro-steroidal hormone that decreases as we age. A decrease in DHEA levels is linked to many degenerative and chronic illnesses like neurological functioning, stress disorders, depression, coronary artery disease, and cancer.

Immunity could have been compromised by poor regulation of cellular hormones that rule immune response due to the aging process.

A dietary approach is worth pursuing. There are many supplements out there and finding the right ones can be hard.

Always consult your doctor before deciding to take supplements to make sure none of them will react with your other medications that may have been prescribed to you. Investigate and explore your options.

CHAPTER 13: EXERCISE

Autoimmune diseases will throw your body off course. Your body is attacking its own tissues. What is normally good for you – like trying to boost the immune system – could actually make things worse. You will have to restrict eating foods that actually are nutrient dense and healthy. You cannot take anything for granted and have to think about and measure everything before you eat it. It may feel as if everything is a trigger.

Does this hold true for exercise as well? Do people who have been diagnosed with autoimmune diseases have to change how they train?

Exercise can actually help. You just need to learn to do it the right way or incur harmful effects.

Try not to overtrain. Many autoimmune diseases have chronic inflammation. Whatever causes this inflammation to increase, like exercising too much, contributes to this pain. Overtraining will increase autoimmune symptoms because it increases your stress load.

Stay away from exercise that induces leaky gut. Intense, protracted exercise like 30 minutes of high-intensity metabolic workouts, 400-meter high-intensity intervals, long runs at race pace, all these will increase intestinal permeability. Leaky gut is linked to ankylosing spondylitis and rheumatoid arthritis. Researchers think it might play a role in hurting other autoimmune diseases, also.

Not exercising can make matters worse since it increases endorphins. Endorphins are actually what the body pumps out when it is trying to deal with pain and as a response to exercise. Exogenous opiates work through the endorphin receptor system. Endorphins play an important role in immune functions. Instead of diminishing or boosting it, endorphins will regulate immunity. They keep the system running smoothly. Without endorphins, the immune system will misbehave. Do this sound familiar?

Low Doses of Naltrexone or LDN is a good therapy for multiple sclerosis or another disease. It increases the endorphin secretions that will help regulate the system's behavior. Exercise is not as effective as LDN, but it does help.

It has the exact same relationship as everybody has when exercising. Too little is bad. Too much is bad. Recovery is a must. Intensity has to be balanced with the volume. When you have an autoimmune disease, the margin of error is a lot smaller.

What's the right way to exercise? It all depends on which autoimmune disease you have. Let's look at some common ones:

Rheumatoid Arthritis

This disease hurts. It makes exercise seem impossible. This is why many who have RA stay inactive. Exercise will help.

Exercise can improve functionality, reduce depression, and improve sleep. Acute exercise will keep cartilage from being destroyed and can help to thicken it.

What will work?

Yoga works. Many RA patients who did yoga regularly benefited from it. Yoga can reduce pain, improve function, and increase general well-being.

Light intensity activities work as well. Studies have shown that about five hours of light intensity activity every day was effective at improving cardiovascular health in RA patients instead of 35 minutes of moderate intensity training every day. This is not unique to RA; everyone can benefit from moving and walking for five hours instead of just jogging for 30 minutes.

Moving the painful joints works. For patients who have finger joint and hand pain, an exercise program that is centered on their hands can help improve functionality.

High-intensity activities will work. Four 4-minute high-intensity intervals on a bike exercise at 85 to 95 percent max rate can increase muscle mass and cardio fitness while reducing inflammatory markers for people who have RA. Patients could perform high-intensity aerobic and resistance training without having any issues.

Multiple Sclerosis

Just like RA, people who have multiple sclerosis can benefit from exercise. They begin to sleep better. If you begin early in life, you could reduce getting MS. Exercise increases brain-derived neurotrophic factors that are reduced in MS.

What works?

Tai Chi works. Tai chi improves functional outcomes in people who have MS.

Endurance and strength training work better together than alone. Doing a 24-week endurance and lifting program can increase BDNF (Brain-derived neurotrophic factor) in MS patients. A 12-week high-intensity and lifting program improved glucose tolerance.

Lifting during the morning works. Studies have shown that MS patients had less muscle strength and more muscle fatigue in the afternoons when compared to morning. Muscle oxidative capacity or the ability to burn fat did not change with times.

Intense exercise works. The higher the intensity, the more BDNF you make. BDNF is essential for creating and maintaining healthy neurons for a healthier brain.

Crohn's Disease

The body will attack the GI tract with Crohn's Disease. Since Crohn's could cause crippling GI pain, emergency diarrhea, joint pain, fatigue, and impaired digestion, many patients avoid exercise. Exercise can actually help a patient if they to overcome their mental roadblocks.

What will work?

Medium-intensity activities and short sprints work. Moderate cycling and all-out cycling were tolerated by children who have been diagnosed with Crohn's. In the moderate group, the markers were high. Another marker stayed elevated longer in the moderate group.

Aerobic and resistance training works. Both or alone will improve Crohn's symptoms by helping immune function.

Walking will work. A low-intensity walk three times each week will improve the quality of life for Crohn's patients.

Type-1 Diabetes

People forget about type-1 diabetes. This autoimmune disease attacks the pancreas and reduces the ability to make insulin. For patients that want to reduce how much insulin they inject, exercise is necessary.

What works?

Combining aerobic and resistance training works. This combination can lower insulin requirements and improve every marker of fitness as well as general feeling.

Resistance training works. Resistance training can lower blood glucose regardless of what intensity. Patients might need a dose of insulin after working out to keep glucose under control.

Lift heavy but keep it brief. High-intensity and low-volume short sprints like three to five rep sets. Intensity is relative so do not try to squat your bodyweight at first.

Spend the time on training on slow, long movements. Gardening walks, hikes, and gentle movements are the best. Anyone who has an autoimmune disease can do these.

Mobility training is needed with a disease that bothers joints and connective tissues. If the joints are compromised, other tissues need to be more mobile, loose, and limber.

Having an autoimmune disease will not make you fragile. You can still exercise if you give your body time to recover.

Find a Support Group

Having an autoimmune disease might leave you feeling isolated and alone. When you have finally processed the diagnosis, finding support from others might help you. Patients who have practical and emotional support during hard times have a handle on emotional health, improved health outcomes, and better quality of life.

If you do not like talking about your illness, you are not the only one. Most people find it hard to talk about their problems.

Why would you need support? You need support especially in the early stages, even if you just reach out to a couple of people. Here is why:

Support reduces stress: Talking about your feelings can reduce your stress. This is important since stress triggers symptoms for most.

Support will keep you on track: Having somebody to check in on you and see that you are taking your meds or eating right can help you control your illness.

You can get help faster in an emergency: If you have a health crisis at home or work, you will get through it if family or friends know how to help.

You will be more stable at work: Symptoms could occur at work and interfere with your job. Telling a co-worker or supervisor that you trust about what is going on can make it easier to continue working in spite of your illness.

How to Build a Support Team

There are many resources out there to help you when you have an illness. Try these:

Journal: You are the most important part of your support team. Write down your ideas, feelings, and thoughts. This is a good way to get rid of stress and plan other ways of communicating about the illness.

Reach out to friends and family: This needs to be your first stop. Be careful how you tell your loved one, so you do not overwhelm them. Do not whine. If you have a complaint, share it in a way to keep people listening.

Become a member of a faith community: For some, being a member of a faith community can give emotional benefits like stress reduction.

Join a support group: Talk to others who are coping with the same illness. They can give you invaluable emotional support and tips.

Go online: People who are limited or isolated with mobility can find help online. Some national foundations and societies support certain chronic illnesses.

Find help for depression: People who have a chronic illness often suffer from depression. Your doctor might prescribe an antidepressant to help with anxiety and depression. If you are feeling suicidal or overwhelmed, seek additional therapy. Depression is a reason to have a support group since isolation can contribute to depression.

Take time to nurture your illness: This will give you invaluable benefits for your emotional health.

CHAPTER 14: MOTIVATION

If you have ever thought about ways you can stay healthy and fit, you may have realized that you are in serious need of motivation. It could be external or internal, but you must wake up each morning and stay motivated through the day and make the right choices when it comes to eating. The foods you eat will help you get through your workouts and will push you to the next level.

When struggling with any chronic illness, it is challenging to stay motivated, or you might be completely passionate. It just depends on your set of mind. Once you have been diagnosed with an autoimmune disease, you might think staying fit is impossible. Many people live the total opposite of healthy and fit. Not because their health problems prevented them from staying healthy and fit but mostly because they think negatively about their well-being.

This is not the case. Many people choose not to benefit from eating healthy and exercising to manage their disease. These people are just too lazy to care about their health. Staying fit is a challenge when you do not even feel like getting out of bed. Being fatigued is not anything to laugh at. It affects how you can handle your daily life.

So can you stay motivated, healthy, and fit when you have an autoimmune disease? Yes.

Begin each day with staying positive. It is hard to stay positive when you are in constant pain. Reminding yourself when you wake up that today is going to be a beautiful day will help substantially.

Promise yourself that you are going to do one thing that your body will thank you for. Feel grateful that you will fight this disease with pride. This is easier when you are in remission. It can motivate you to get out of bed and choice a healthy food for breakfast or take a walk.

Make smart food choices. It is not easy to eat right when everybody around you is eating burgers and fries. Bad food is your enemy. Eating the wrong foods is the quickest way to flare up your condition. You have to be extremely smart about food choices. Learn your body and know what it can and cannot handle. If you do not want to wake up in pain the next day, make smart food choices today. This might seem too easy for people who want to be fit, but it is a true challenge for individuals with an autoimmune disease. One bad food choice can cause pain for weeks. Just don't do it. Learn to love your body and give it the food it needs and what it can handle.

You will fuse if you do not move. This is a great reminder for anyone who suffers from arthritis, but it holds true for any autoimmune disease. Just move. Your body is going to thank you. It does not have to be at an extremely intense movement. Just walk or do some low-intensity weight training a couple of times a week. Make sure you move. Try to do it for 30 minutes for about three or four days each week. When you begin to feel stronger, your body will amaze you on how it responds. You could get healthier from exercising alone, and it's great.

Know that you are going to have bad days. Do not get discouraged. There are going to be bad days. You will have days that you will not be able to eat or exercise right at all. The main thing here is to never give up. Accept that your body is going to win every now and then and you just need to listen to it and rest. Love yourself and learn to listen to your body. There will be other days that you can exercise. Tomorrow is just one day away. You will get active soon.

Learn to love your body. Listen to your body. Feed it with real, bountiful, and beautiful foods. Push it a bit so you can begin to feel better. Acknowledge and listen when you might be pushing it too far. Make health and fitness a priority and your body will start thanking you.

CHAPTER 15: FOOD LIST

To help you get started in changing the way you eat to help your autoimmune disease, this chapter will provide you with a list of the best foods to consume.

Fruits and Vegetables

- All types of vegetables with lots of variety
- Colorful fruits and vegetables
- Cruciferous vegetables
- Sea vegetables – excluding algae
- Watercress
- Turnips
- Mustard greens
- Kale
- Cabbage

- Brussels sprouts

- Broccoli

- Arugula

Fruits and Vegetables to Avoid

- Tomatillos

- Tamarillos

- Potatoes – sweet potatoes

- Pimentos

- Pepinos

- Paprika

- Naranjillas

- Kutjera

- Hot peppers – habanero jalapenos

- Goji berries

- Garden huckleberry

- Eggplant

- Cocona

- Capsicum

- Cape gooseberry

- Bush tomato

- Ashwagandha

Protein

- Glycine-rich foods

- Fish and shellfish

- Offal and organ meat

- Wild boar

- Venison

- Turkey – in moderation

- Rabbit

- Pork

- Pheasant – in moderation

- Lamb

- Elk

- Duck – in moderation

- Chicken – in moderation

- Buffalo

- Beef

Fats

- Olives
- Animal fats
- Fatty fish
- Coconut
- Avocados

Probiotics

- Water and coconut milk kefir
- Kombucha
- Fermented fruits and veggies
- Coconut milk yogurt

Spices and herbs

- Turmeric
- Thyme
- Tarragon
- Spearmint
- Savory leaves
- Salt
- Sage
- Saffron
- Rosemary

- Peppermint
- Parsley
- Oregano leaves
- Onion powder
- Marjoram leaves
- Mace
- Lavender
- Horseradish
- Ginger
- Garlic
- Dill weed
- Cloves
- Cinnamon
- Coriander
- Chives
- Chervil
- Chamomile
- Bay leaves
- Basil
- Lemon balm

Spices and Herbs to eat in moderation

- White pepper

- Vanilla bean

- Star anise

- Pink peppercorns

- Juniper

- Green peppercorns

- Cardamom

- Caraway

- Black pepper

- Allspice

Spices and herbs to avoid

- Sesame seed

- Poppy seed

- Paprika

- Nutmeg

- Mustard seed

- Fenugreek

- Fennel seed

- Dill seed

- Cumin seeds

- Curry

- Coriander seeds

- Chili powder

- Chili pepper flakes

- Celery seeds

- Cayenne

- Black caraway

- Annatto seed

- Anise seed

Other foods that need to be avoided

- Seeds – seed-based spices, coffee, cocoa

- Nuts

- NSAIDs – ibuprofen or aspirin

- Non-nutritive sweeteners – stevia

- Fructose – no more than 20g each day

- Food additives

- Thickeners and emulsifiers

- Eggs – especially the whites

- Alcohol

Foods which cross-react with gluten

- Teff

- Tapioca

- Soy

- Spelt

- Sorghum

- Sesame

- Rye

- Rice

- Quinoa

- Potato

- Polish wheat

- Oats

- Milk

- Millet

- Hemp

- Corn

- Coffee – imported, espresso, latte, instant

- Chocolate

- Buckwheat

- Barley

- amaranth

For the grains, you can select what kind of grain you want. But always remember, when choosing food, you should go by how certain food makes you feel. You may be able to eat something that another person cannot. This is just a guideline; the important thing is just to get to know you.

PART 5:

MEAL PLAN AND RECIPES

CHAPTER 16: MEAL PLAN

To help get you started with your autoimmune diet, in this section, you will find a one-week meal plan and the recipes that correspond with it. These are fun and tasty recipes, and an extremely easy meal plan to stick to. You will be making most of what you will eat all week on Sunday. One recipe, the Bacon-Beef Liver Pate is for a snack during the week. Let's get started.

Sunday:

- Breakfast: Italian-Spiced 50/50 Sausages
- Lunch: Cabbage and Avocado Salad

- Dinner: Citrus and Herb Pot Roast and Rainbow Roasted Root Vegetables

Monday:

- Breakfast: Three-Herb Beef Patties
- Lunch: Citrus and Herb Pot Roast and Rainbow Roasted Root Vegetables
- Dinner: Citrus and Herb Pot Roast and Cabbage and Avocado Salad

Tuesday:

- Breakfast: Italian-Spiced 50/50 Sausages
- Lunch: Citrus and Herb Pot Roast and Rainbow Roasted Root Vegetables
- Dinner: Ginger-Baked Salmon and Beet and Fennel Salad

Wednesday:

- Breakfast: Three-Herb Beef Patties
- Lunch: Ginger Baked Salmon and Beet and Fennel Salad

- Dinner: Carrot and Sweet Potato Chili

Thursday:

- Breakfast: Italian-Spiced 50/50 Sausages
- Lunch: Carrot and Sweet Potato Chili
- Dinner: Sear-Roasted Pork Chops and Early Spring Salad

Friday:

- Breakfast: Three-Herb Beef Patties
- Lunch: Sear-Roasted Pork Chops and Early Spring Salad
- Dinner: Carrot and Sweet Potato Chili

Saturday:

- Breakfast: Italian-Spiced 50/50 Sausages
- Lunch: Carrot and Sweet Potato Chili
- Dinner: Garlic Mayo Shredded Chicken Breast Curried Chicken Salad

Cabbage and Avocado Salad

Ingredients:

2 cubed avocados

3 tsp. salt

2 tsp. coconut vinegar

4 tbsps. olive oil

2 blood oranges, juiced

1 handful parsley, chopped

3 carrots, grated

1 small red onion, sliced

1 head cabbage, shredded

Instructions:

Toss together the carrots, onion, cabbage, and most of the parsley.

Mix the salt, coconut vinegar, olive oil, and the orange

juice.

Pour the dressing over the vegetables and toss together.

Add the remaining parsley and the avocado on top.

Citrus and Herb Pot Roast

Ingredients:

Fresh herbs

2 parsnips, chunked

3 carrots, chunked

1 bay leaf

1 orange, juiced

2 tbsps. Apple Cider Vinegar (ACV)

¾ c bone broth

1 ½ tsp. salt

2-3 lbs. roast

1 tbsp. coconut oil

Instructions:

Your oven should be at 300 F. Add the coconut oil into a Dutch oven and then place in the roast and brown it on all sides. Turn the heat off and take the roast out of the pot and salt it.

Place the bay leaf, orange juice, cider vinegar, and bone broth into the pot. Place the roast back in and surround it with the parsnips and carrots. Add a generous sprinkling of the fresh herbs over everything.

Cover the pot with a lid and place it in the oven for two to three hours. Make sure that you check to make sure there is enough liquid in the pot every now and then. Once cooked, pull the meat apart with some forks and enjoy.

Rainbow Roasted Root Vegetables

Ingredients:

1 tsp. salt

3 tbsps. coconut oil

2 parsnips, chunked

3 carrots, chunked

1 turnip, chunked

4 beets, chunked

Instructions:

Your oven should be at 400 F. Mix together the parsnip, carrots, turnip, and beets together and place them on a baking sheet. Sprinkle with some salt and drizzle with some melted coconut oil.

Place them in the oven and cook for 45 to 60 minutes. Make sure you stir every 20 minutes so that everything becomes tender and caramelized.

Ginger Baked Salmon

Ingredients:

3 tbsps. parsley, minced

¼ tsp. sea salt

¼ tsp. ginger

2 tbsps. melted coconut oil

16/24 oz. salmon fillet

Instructions:

Your oven should be at 400 F. Clean your salmon and place it onto an oiled baking sheet. Rush the coconut oil over the fillet and sprinkle it with sea salt and ginger. Place in the oven for 15 to 20 minutes.

Beet and Fennel Salad

Ingredients:

Dressing:

¼ tsp. salt

1 minced garlic clove

½ lemon, juiced

1 tbsp. ACV

½ c olive oil

Salad:

Sprig mint, chopped

Handful parsley, chopped

1 fennel bulb

1 cucumber

4 beets

Instructions

Mix all of the dressing ingredients in a bowl. Slice up the fennel, beets, and cucumber very thinly. Add them to a large bowl and toss them together with the dressing.

Carrot and Sweet Potato Chili

Ingredients:

Cilantro

1-2 avocados

2 lbs. ground beef

1 tsp. salt

4 c bone broth

4 c sweet potatoes, chunked

2 c carrots, chunked

1 tbsp. thyme

8 minced garlic cloves

1 onion, chopped

2 tbsps. coconut oil

Instructions:

Melt the coconut oil in a large pot. Place in the onion and allow to cook until soft, and then mix in the thyme and garlic, cooking for a few more minutes.

Place the sweet potato and carrot and let them cook for about five minutes. Pour in the salt and the bone broth and allow it to come to a boil. Place on the lid and let cook for 20 minutes. Veggies should be soft.

Add in the ground beef and mix. Let it cook for another 15 minutes. Serve with a slice of avocado and cilantro.

Italian-spiced 50/50 sausages

Ingredients:

1 tbsp. coconut oil

½ tsp. salt

½ tsp. garlic powder

1 tbsp. minced parsley

1 tbsp. minced thyme

1 tbsp. minced oregano

1 lb. ground pork

1 lb. ground beef

Instructions:

Add all of the ingredients, except for the oil, in a bowl
and mix them with your hands until well combined.
Form the meat into eight to ten patties. You can
freeze them now by placing wax paper between the

patties and sliding them into a freezer safe bag or container.

When you are ready to eat, melt the oil and fry them for 10 minutes per side.

Three-Herb Beef Patties

Ingredients:

1 tbsp. coconut oil

1 tsp. salt

1 tbsp. sage

1 tbsp. thyme

1 tbsp. rosemary

2 lbs. ground beef

Instructions:

Mix all of the herbs, beef, and salt together with your hands. Form them into patties. At this point, they can be frozen with wax paper between the patties.

Once ready to cook them, heat the oil in a skillet and fry for about five to eight minutes on each side.

Bacon-Beef Liver Pate

Ingredients:

1/2 tsp. salt

½ c melted coconut oil

2 tbsps. thyme, minced

2 tbsps. rosemary, minced

1 lb. beef liver

4 minced garlic cloves

1 onion, minced

6 pcs. bacon

Instructions:

Cook the bacon until it is crisp and allow to cool.
Place the onion in the bacon grease and let cook for
two minutes. Mix in the garlic and add the liver.

Sprinkle everything with herbs and let cook for three to five minutes or until cooked through.

Turn the heat off and add everything to a blender and mix with the coconut oil and salt until it turns into a paste.

Cut the bacon up and stir it into the plate.

Sear-Roasted Pork Chops

Ingredients:

1 tbsp. coconut oil

1 tsp. salt

2 tbsps. fresh herbs

2 pork chops

Instructions:

Your oven should be at 350 F. Mix the salt and herbs together. Add oil to a pan, and then rub the herbs over the chops.

Once the pan is hot, sear the chops for a couple of minutes on each side. Slide them into the oven for ten minutes.

Early Spring Salad

Ingredients:

1 fennel bulb, sliced

1 grapefruit, sectioned

4 c arugula

¼ tsp. salt

¼ tsp. ginger

1 tbsp. ACV

1 lemon, juiced

¼ c EVOO

Instructions:

Add the salt, ginger, vinegar, lemon juice, and olive oil in a bowl and mix well.

Add the all the other ingredients into the bowl and toss together. Toss with the dressing just before serving.

Garlic Mayo

Ingredients:

¼ tsp. salt

3-4 garlic cloves

¼ c EVOO

½ c warm water

½ c coconut concentrate, warmed

Instructions:

Place the salt, garlic, olive oil, water, and coconut in a blender and mix until the sauce thickens.

Allow this to cool to room temp.

Curried Chicken Salad

Ingredients:

2 tbsps. parsley, chopped

¼ c raisins

¼ c chopped onion

1 lb. chicken breast, cooked and shredded

¼ tsp. salt

1 tsp. ginger

2 tsp. turmeric

½ lemon, juiced

1 tsp. ACV

½ c garlic mayo

Instructions:

Whisk together the salt, ginger, turmeric, lemon juice, vinegar, and mayo. Mix in the raisins, onion, and chicken. Serve with some parsley.

CONCLUSION

Thank you for making it through to the end of *Power Over Autoimmune.* Let's hope it was informative and able to provide you with all of the tools you need to achieve your goals.

Throughout this book, you have learned a lot of information about autoimmune diseases, and many ways to approach them. Next, you need to start trying these practices. Pick what works best for you and reverse your autoimmune disease.

Just because you have an autoimmune disease or condition does not mean you have to suffer from all of the symptoms and other problems associated with it. You can make changes to improve the quality of your life.

Again, if you found this book useful in any way, please do leave a review to help me get the word out to as many people as possible!

All the best to you and your endeavors, and I hope to see you soon!

Best,

Gregg Haven M.D.